I0420912

12 Essential Oils for Natural Weight Loss

The Ultimate Beginner's Guide To Feeling Better With Aromatherapy

William J. Walker

© 2015

Disclaimer

All rights reserved. No part of this publication may be reproduced, distributed, or transmitted in any form or by any means, including photocopying, recording, or other electronic or mechanical methods, without the prior written permission of the publisher, except in the case of brief quotations embodied in critical reviews and certain other noncommercial uses permitted by copyright law.

This book is not intended as a substitute for the medical advice of physicians. The reader should regularly consult a physician in matters relating to his/her health and particularly with respect to any symptoms that may require diagnosis or medical attention.

TABLE OF CONTENTS

Introduction

Many ancient civilizations, such as the ancestors of modern day Egyptians, Chinese and Indians, as well as, civilizations that have since vanished such as the Romans, understood and in many cases continue to understand and appreciate the therapeutic effects of essential oils. The wisdom of these cultures, unfortunately, has been written off by the closed minded as superstition or witchcraft or completely ineffectual as people instead turn to over marketed drugs produced by pharmaceutical companies who tell people that everything that they feel is not quite right with them, is really an illness and they must take expensive drugs to be healthy and live a fulfilling life.

Rather than helping people, many of these drugs create dependence and have terrible side effects. Despite the fact that doctors and pharmacists are required to notify patients of these side effects, few people actually read the 1500 word hands outs about all of the terrible things that the drugs can do to you. Instead, they trust their doctor or pharmacist to just do what's best. This is in no way a criminalization of doctors and pharmacists, as my parents actually happen to be a doctor and a pharmacist. While there are bad apples in any profession, most such individuals are good people who went into Medicine to help people and they continue to help people. However, while one should never stop taking medicine prescribed by a doctor, there are often better and less expensive alternatives that take a whole body approach to health and have little to no side effects.

Essential oils are among these "drugs" that you do not have to have a prescription to buy, because they are generally safe, when used appropriately. These oils do not pump you full of those harmful chemicals that our bodies often reject; rather they work naturally, the way nature intended. They work with our bodies and not against them. They do not artificially stimulate various glands and systems; instead they nurture our organs so that we can function at our peak. They improve our overall health, aid in digestion, boost our metabolism, regenerate our tissue and help our body absorb more vitamins and minerals. Essential oils are not the "magic pill" for fast weight loss or fast anything. They are so much more than that as they are help us at the cellular level. They help us get started on our way to healthier, fitter bodies and stronger minds. They don't affect only our body, but our psyche as well, helping us find balance and improve our mood. Essential oils are a whole new world for you to discover and this is a helpful guide for you in which I will introduce some of the most used essential oils for weight loss. If you have to make a choice between taking some pills for "fast weight loss" and taking a slow, but safe ride with natural ingredients, go natural. It is far safer and much healthier.

When individuals are struggling with their weight, it is not just about food and exercise, as some might believe. Yes, calories in-calories out is an effective way to lose weight, but it is often only temporary because you are not actually addressing why you are eating too many calories or not getting enough exercise. You are thinking of the effect and not the cause. When our bodies are not properly in balance, we are hungry all the time, we are tired and we often neglect doing those things we love, with those we love simply due to lack of energy.

The information presented in this book about essential oils and their many benefits is not meant to be an end all or some sort of quick fix for weight loss or whatever things may be ailing you. Rather they should open your eyes to the value that can be added to your life by simply incorporating one or few of these oils into your daily routine as they work to make you better from the inside out. Incorporating these oils should help to provide balance; mental, physical and spiritual balance. When these things are in balance you will find yourself having a better relationship with food and its intended function, which is nourishment, and not as comfort food or something to do to help past the time.

So enough with all of that let's dive in and explore together how essential oils can help you be a healthier, fitter, naturally better you.

Chapter 1

Grapefruit Oil

Grapefruit essential oil is in the top-three essential oils for weight loss. It looks nice, smells nice and is tasty, but most people aren't aware how powerful this citrus is and how it can help us burn more fat and lose serious weight. Let me start by saying that if you are on any prescription medications, especially birth control or antibiotics be careful when consuming grapefruit oil as it can alter the way the drug was intended to perform. That is not something to be afraid but simply read the warning labels on any medications prescribed or ask your physician to be 100 percent certain. Grapefruit oil is a powerful essential oil. You may already be saying, yuck! I hate grapefruit. Maybe this book isn't for me. If you are, please bear with me a moment, so I can make one thing clear. When it comes to essential oils, the amount needed to have the desired effect will be minimal and typically diffused in oil, inhaled, rubbed on, etc. So even if you would normally not eat a whole grapefruit or even a half of one, you can still appreciate and use this essential oil and reap its many benefits.

What makes grapefruit so powerful? Grapefruit peel contains a compound called D-limonene, which can be also found in other citrus fruits in various potencies. This compound reacts with enzymes in our body and causes a decrease of appetite, more efficient fat burning and it is great for our immune system.

Grapefruit oil is an antioxidant, disinfectant, antiseptic, antidepressant, diuretic and it contributes to weight loss. This fruit can really be a miracle for your body and over time, with regular use, the effects can be amazing.

Cleansing our body is the first step in weight loss. You cannot expect a dirty machine to perform at maximum capacity or even mediocre capacity for that matter. Our body is just like a machine, very delicate and sensitive to abuse and will ultimately breakdown if not taken care of and serviced regularly. Eating healthy foods and watching sugar intake can improve energy levels and promote optimum performance. Incorporating grapefruit oil can reduce the frequency in which you get colds while revitalizing your immune system. You will have more strength and you may find yourself being in an overall better mood. Grapefruit is packed with vitamin c, and it's well known that vitamin c is crucial for detoxification and cleansing our body. Vitamin C with other compounds found in the grapefruit peel are key to a strong immune system. The improved lymphatic function that citrus can provide is probably its best asset. The lymphatic system has the most important role in the body, as it is responsible for removing all the harmful waste that frankly does our body no good and works to regenerate our bodies from the inside out.

If you are like most people, you eat and drink and come in contact with lots of junk that may taste good but ultimately it doesn't promote our bodies to perform as well as they should and could. Our bodies have to remove this stuff from our cells or it weighs us down leaving us fat and tired and not functioning as nature intended. When we use things like Grapefruit oil to help our lymphatic system more efficiently detoxify, our body is working as it should and stubborn weight just can't hold on any more. This is in no way saying that grapefruit oil somehow negates the effects of ice cream, cookies and beer. Rather it is encourages your body to appropriately dispose of the toxins found in these food choices so that our bodies are freed up to perform the functions of living. This leaves us feeling more energetic and youthful.

Grapefruit oil has a significant influence on our digestive system as it stimulates the secretion of gastric juices and helps aid in digestion of food as well as the movement of ingested food through the intestines. Many believe that consuming acidic foods like grapefruit are key contributors to digestive issues like acid reflux, indigestion and even ulcers, but to the contrary, our body needs acid. It's what our stomach is filled with. Acid is what digests food. When we are having these issues with digestion, our bodies are actually telling us that we need more acidic foods in our diet. Regularly using grapefruit oil helps maintain that acid balance in your stomach, which means better digestion, which leads to better absorption of vitamins and minerals so that our bodies remain in homeostasis and we can lose those unwanted pounds. Grapefruit oil can also help to decrease your appetite, and can help to curb cravings.

As if the benefits listed already weren't enough grapefruit oil is great for keeping your skin clean and acne-free. It can help heal various skin ailments and prevent future problems. Many anti-cellulite creams have grapefruit essential oil as one of the main ingredients because it is an excellent diuretic and healthy lymphatic stimulant.

How To Use Grapefruit Oil?

Add 1-2 drops to your glass of water. Water will help flush those unwanted, unhelpful toxins out. For best results, you should have a glass of warm water with a few drops before your breakfast. It will burn fat more efficiently since your stomach is empty, and warm water will improve digestion.

Applying grapefruit oil directly to those "problematic" areas is another great use. Mix a few drops of grapefruit oil into ½ oz. of organic virgin coconut oil or extra virgin olive oil. Massage it into skin until fully absorbed.

If you like long soothing baths add five drops or so to a warm bath and enjoy aromatherapy at home. It's great for soothing your mind, and warm water will open up pores so the skin can absorb the grapefruit oil better allowing you to reap the benefits inside and out.

Chapter 2

Ginger Oil

If you ever googled "drinks that help weight loss" you must have come across the recipe for a ginger lemonade. It is one of the most common recipes given to boost your metabolism, strengthen your immune system and help you shed a few pounds. Ginger has compounds called gingerols that help your body absorb more vitamins (like vitamin C in lemon) and minerals. It is like your body is an upscale nightclub with a special VIP entrance in the back and you have to know the password to get in. Regardless of how famous this VIP is or how much money the nightclub knows that VIP will spend, if they don't know the password, they are not getting in no matter what. Many vitamins and minerals that your body must have to function are like these VIPs that we are rejecting because they don't know the password to get in. Did you know that even when you eat super healthy foods, your body might be absorbing less than a quarter of the nutrition from those foods? That is really disappointing when you are trying to do good things for your body, and it is especially bad if you are only eating super healthy foods like raw veggies, fruits, nuts, seeds and omega-3 containing oils a few times a week. Over time it leads to sluggishness, weight gain, moodiness and poor health. It's like vitamins and minerals need the combination to our bodies, a special access code to enter our bodies effectively. Otherwise these VIPs, called vitamins and minerals, are treated like waste that our body needs to remove with all of the excess sugar and heavy metals we ingest. Ginger, with its healthy gingerols, is their password, which allows vitamins and minerals to not be treated as unwanted guests, but like the VIPs they are, who are welcomed with open arms, given the special treatment and access to wherever they want to go in your body. And vitamins and minerals know where to go once they get inside. They are going to go where they are needed most to keep you running like a well oiled machine. This analogy helps us understand why ginger oil is such a good oil for weight loss – with more vitamins and minerals absorbed, your body will have more cellular energy, and it will burn fat more efficiently. It is as easy as that.

If you have sugar cravings often, ginger oil will reduce your cravings, and it helps you turn the sugar you consumed into energy instead of having it sitting in your body and eventually becoming excess weight on your hips, thighs and midsection. When we are actually using the sugar that comes into our bodies, this means that we are not giving it an opportunity to turn into fat storage, which is ultimately where all unburned energy ends up, regardless of how healthy that original source of energy was.

Ginger is also highly efficient in fighting Candida (yeast overgrowth in intestines due to high sugar intake and weak immune system). Candida are some of the most evil little you-know-what's that ever existed. Candida are living organisms that live inside your body, in other words, parasites. Having some candida in your system is okay and perfectly natural, but when you have too much, some very bad things happen to your body inside and out. It can manifest itself in different ways in different people, but for most, overgrowth will cause headaches, fatigue, cravings and even very serious skin problems like the inability of the skin to heal as well as scaling, skin ulcers, dryness, psoriasis, dermatitis and eczema. Pretty bad stuff, right? If you have ever suffered from severe skin problems you know how they can control your life. While, some people are genetically predisposed to certain skin ailments, even they can significantly reduce the effects of the disease and the hold it has on their lives through eliminating candida with ginger oil.

Candida is no joke and you do not want to let it take over your body. One of the reasons that I say it is "evil" is because candida is a survivor. In a zombie apocalypse, you better believe that Candida is the one who knows how to fortify, scavenge and hit that zombie right in the head. It knows how to get what it wants at any cost to continue to thrive and reproduce. If Candida is already overgrown in your system, Candida actually tricks our bodies into thinking that we need to eat more sugar, the primary food source of Candida. When it's 3pm and you feel like you are just going to die if you don't run to the vending machine to get a snickers, this may not actually be you wanting candy at all, and rather it is Candida saying that you need to eat more sugar, not because you need it or really want it, although you may disagree at the time, because the craving is very real, but because the Candida wants more sugar, so that it can multiply in your system and wreak more havoc on your body and your life.

Ginger is like that friend who always has your back and says, "No, Candida, you are not going to treat my friend like that. My friend deserves better and you will not control him or her." Your best bud, Ginger defends you against Candida overgrowth, which stops those "fake" cravings and the side effects that the sugar and the Candida overgrowth cause to our system.

Ginger is like that shoulder to lean on. She is there for you as long as you invite her over regularly. She is going to help you battle cravings, get the nutrients you need and feel fuller longer because she's got things under control.

How To Use Ginger Oil?

Like mentioned before, add a few drops to a cup of hot/warm water with lemon. You can add honey if you want to have a healthy desert.

There are several ways you can inhale ginger oil. You can inhale directly from the bottle, or you can put a few drops on a cloth and inhale it that way. Another inhalation way is putting a few drops on your palms. Whatever works for you. Ginger oil is used for soothing tired and tensed muscles. For muscle relief rub a few drops of oil on the part aching and massage it into skin thoroughly. Ginger oil also helps with digestion. For digestion problems, you should rub a few drops on your stomach and gently massage it. You can get creative and make DIY aromatherapy candles: take your old candles and cut them into pieces (take out the wick), take a large cooking pot, about a ½ cup of water and heat the water until boiling. Take one smaller pot, put it over the heated water (so-called water steam melting) and put pieces of the candle inside, wait until they melt down and add essential oil. Stir it and pour into a candle pot, insert the wick and wait for it to become solid. Enjoy your aromatherapy candle.

Chapter 3

Cinnamon Oil

The Cinnamon spice we use is derived from inner bark or leaves of the tree Cinnamomum. Cinnamon is used widely for health and flavoring purposes. When not using cinnamon on your favorite desert or treat, use cinnamon to help regulate blood glucose levels and help with glucose tolerance.

How can cinnamon oil help in weight loss? Cinnamon is great for suppressing sugar cravings. One of the reasons we crave sugar, other than the Candida, which we discussed in the last chapter, is due to a low level of sugar in our blood. Cinnamon helps stabilize blood sugar, so that it does not get too high, leading to headaches, nervousness and dizziness and it does not get to low, leading to light-headedness, fatigue and sugar cravings. When you consume cinnamon, glucose is released at a slower rate, helping blood sugar levels stabilize.

Our blood sugar can be like a rollercoaster, going up and down. When we are at a theme park, this movement between extremes can leave us feeling terrible and looking for the nearest trashcan. It's the same thing with blood sugar, as allowing it to get too high or too low over and over makes us really sick and can even lead to really bad things like type 2 diabetes. Unfortunately, in our busy lives we often turn to sugar filled processed foods for quick nourishment because who has time to cook or prepare healthy whole food meals from scratch any more, this means that we are sending our blood sugar shooting to the top of that rollercoaster and then, because sugar is a simple form of energy and doesn't stay sugar for long (it turns to fat) we are sailing back down to the bottom of the coaster at which time we start craving more sugar and we start the cycle again and again. This leads to poor food choices because when you are in hunger/craving mode you just want something that tastes good and it can seem impossible to resist.

Cinnamon is like your other BFF who is always there to bring you stability. When you start going off the deep end in one direction or the other, your levelheaded friend, Cinnamon is the one who brings you balance, so you don't go quite so high or fall so low that it makes you sick. Cinnamon does this by regulating insulin in the blood and helping your body convert blood glucose into energy by boosting your metabolism, so that you are not storing it as fats.

Cinnamon oil also improves digestion. Some refer to cinnamon oil as the digestive tonic because it has many positive effects on your digestive system: it reduces the feeling of flatulence, by eliminating excess gas from your stomach and intestines, and it fights diarrhea and vomiting because it is a regulator of your systems - a pretty nice friend to keep around.

How To Use Cinnamon Oil?

Cinnamon is often found in recipes with ginger, lemon, and honey. You can add a drop or two in your morning glass of water with lemon and ginger essential oil. Add some honey for a sweet pleasure. This combination is great at detoxication and reducing inflammations.

Just like other essential oils, you can inhale it from a cotton ball or a soft cloth. You can drink it with water and honey in the morning or before meals since it gives the sense of fullness (30mins before, not less because your stomach acid will be too diluted and your digestion will be weighted).

Chapter 4

Peppermint Oil

Some of us only think of peppermint as an ingredient in candy canes. You may be asking yourself, "Are you going to say candy canes are good for me? Let me answer that one from the start, no. While most things are okay in moderation, candy canes have a lot of sugar and therefore are not something you should be eating regularly to get the benefit of peppermint. There are better alternatives that still taste great, but first let's talk about benefits.

Some refer to peppermint oil as an digestive aid, due to its benefits for your intestines and stomach. Peppermint soothes an upset stomach, and it is very helpful with digestive problems. Peppermint has menthol, which has a calming and cooling effect. It is the most common ingredient of muscle relief gels and creams because this is one of the few essential oils that really gets the respect it deserves from the medical community. Studies have shown that peppermint is highly efficient as an appetite suppressant, and, when used regularly, it lowers hunger levels, so people consume significantly fewer calories.

Peppermint oil can be a great alternative to caffeine consumption as it contains up to 70% menthol which can help increase levels of alertness, raise energy levels and combat fatigue, all while not having the addiction potential like caffeine. How can this help you lose weight? You will have more energy for your workouts, you will work out longer ad/or harder, and you will burn more calories. Peppermint is like a motivational coach. There reminding you that you can do it if you just push a little harder and work just a little longer, but Peppermint is not all talk. He is there, giving you the tools you need, like energy and reduced appetite, so that you can be successful at staying healthy and losing weight.

How To Use Peppermint Oil?

If you want to have more energy during your workouts, apply a few drops on your wrist and inhale it once in a while for a more alert state of body and mind. One of the ways to use peppermint essential oil is to make DIY mouth freshener. Simply mix a few drops of peppermint oil with water in a small glass spray bottle, shake it well and you have your peppermint spray that you can use to curb hunger cravings or simply to refresh your mouth.

Just like any other essential oil, you can put a few drops a warm bath and let peppermint oil get inside your body through your now open pores. Inhaling peppermint oil every 2-4 hours can be another highly effective way to keep you feeling satisfied and discourages overeating and excessive snacking between meals.

Peppermint oil is also amazing when added to hot tea. This way you get the benefits of inhaling and ingesting at the same time, so indulge yourself with a cup instead of giving into cravings. Mint, in general, is also natural treatment option for anxiety. So if you are someone who consumes extra calories when you are anxious, drinking infused tea will calm you right down without making you sleepy.

Chapter 5

Bergamot Oil

Bergamot is another fruit of the citrus family, and just like its other citrus fellows, it has many beneficial compounds in the peel. What makes Bergamot different from other citruses is an extremely large amount of polyphenols, which are antioxidants that halt the production of fat in the blood, which can lead to blood clots and poor circulation. It boosts the metabolism and prevents the absorption of LDL (bad cholesterol).

Lavender, peppermint, and bergamot have one thing in common – they stimulate the endocrine system, helping us feel more relaxed and calm. How can this help your weight loss? Bearing in mind that stress is one of the most common reasons for overeating ("comfort eating"), using some of these essential oils will help us get rid of this bad habit. Emotional eating is the worst kind of overeating because as long as we are under stress, we will continue to overeat and become overweight. The solution is to find the cause of this emotional overeating or to eliminate the stress. Using essential oils helps soothe the mind and find balance. Bergamot is that person in your life, your mom, dad, brother or maybe a significant other, who always lets you know that everything is going to be alright.

Bergamot oil lowers blood sugars and triglycerides; it reduces LDL (bad cholesterol) in the blood and increases the HDL (good cholesterol) percentage in our blood. This means that the highways of our bodies, the blood vessels, are allowing blood cells to move freely at the speed limit or maybe a little over to get where they are going so that it can deliver nutrients and oxygen to our various systems.

As mentioned before, drastically changing blood sugar levels cause sugar cravings and bergamot, like cinnamon, makes sure our blood sugar levels are well balanced.

How To Use Bergamot Oil?

Use bergamot oil for bringing peace and balance to your life. Diffuse a few drops in a pot with water and put it on your working desk or in the living room, whenever you spend the most time. You can make Bergamot aromatherapy candles like mentioned before. Add a few drops to your tea or add a few drops to you face cream for cleaner skin. You can also massage one or two drops of bergamot oil on your stomach to aid in digestion.

Chapter 6

Lemon Oil

Great citrus fruits strike again. Lemon oil with D-Limonene has a similar effect on our body as Grapefruit. Lemon oil is packed with vitamins and minerals, especially vitamin C. Lemon has compounds that help fight intestinal parasites, including, but not limited to Candida, that are often the cause of weight gain. One of the best things you can do for your body is to start your day with a glass of warm lemon water. Add a few drops to a glass of water and drink it every morning. You can combine lemon oil with cinnamon oil and ginger oil. Add some honey, if you prefer a sweeter taste. Lemon water will flush the toxins from your body, it will balance your metabolism, and it will boost your system to maximum performance. Your body will burn more fat, as the cells will be released of toxins and there will be more energy for fat burning. Lemon acid is extremely powerful and can melt down a styrofoam cup, but it has this diffusing effect only on toxic matter and won't harm your body, although, if you are consuming it without significant diffusion, I would drink a glass of water afterwards, so that acid is not sitting on your teeth, which can over time, destroy enamel and lead to cavities.

Use it daily for best results and to keep your body toxin-free. This amazing fruit contains up to 70% of that wonderful D-limonene and its peel is a fat-killer. Lemon oils are added to food in order to protect it against human pathogens such as Escherichia coli (e. Coli-No wonder we always abbreviate it) and Salmonella. Apples and other fruits that tend to brown are often sprayed with lemon juice to prevent the browning and slow the rotting process significantly because bacteria cannot co-exist with lemon. Lemon is like your compulsive cleaner. She likes everything pristine and if no one else is going to do it, she is going to make sure it gets done by doing it herself. Lemon is a well-known natural cleanser for just about every surface. Not only does it disinfect, but it also inhibits the ability of bacteria to live and grow for a significant time after it is used on a surface. It does the same thing for your body.

How To Use Lemon Oil?

Apply and massage a few drops to areas with cellulite. Cellulite is toxins in our cells and by massaging the oil, you will help it get through to cells with toxins and cleanse the cells fast and effectively. This may lead to reducing your thigh volume, for example, because toxins make our cells inflated and cause water retention.

Like mentioned before, drink lemon water. It is the best for detoxifying. It will also reduce your appetite and you will consume fewer calories. Inhaling lemon oil before meals will have the same effect of reducing appetite. You can diffuse few drops in a pot with water and keep it around you for keeping your mind alert and your thoughts clear and focused.

Cleanse surfaces with lemon infused cleaners. Not only are you cleaning, but you are also making your home smell amazing while reaping the benefits of aromatherapy.

Lemon zest is made by scraping the peel of the lemon to release the oils into your food. This is a great way to add a little l-limonene to a salad or other food. Lemon peel, unlike orange peel, can actually be juiced because it is not bitter. Consider juicing a whole lemon every once in a while to feel fantastic.

Chapter 7

Sandalwood Oil

Sandalwood oil has a similar effect on our body and mind as Bergamot oil: it is great for reducing stress levels. Therefore, it's a solution if your problem is stress eating. The wood-like smell is mild and is great for relaxation. Sandalwood scent is often used for incense sticks and candles, and is widely used for meditation and aromatherapy.

What's so amazing with all essential oils is you can be as creative as you want: make candles, make spray diffusers and room fresheners, soak, sprinkle and enjoy. Weight loss has everything to do with your mindset. If your mind is telling you, "you will never lose weight", that is what will happen. If your mind tells you, "you will make it and lose 10 or 20 or 50 pounds", you will. It is all about the way you think and what's crucial to our way of thinking is our stress level. If we are under stress, we will be negative, panicky and over stimulated in a bad way. When we are feeling this way, our body will react just like this, through the process of psycho-somatic (mind-body) response. This is why mental things like stress can cause heart problems, high blood pressure, overeating, ulcers and even strokes and heart attacks. In some current studies that will need to continue to become conclusive, they are even finding strong links between the mental state and the likelihood of getting cancer as well as the chances of surviving cancer. Our mind is affecting our body's ability to function as it should, and the results are devastating if our mind is in turmoil. When we can use essential oils like sandalwood to say "no" to stress the way that people said, "say 'no' to drugs" in the 80's, you are allowing your body to do what it is intended to do and this means efficient use of food and exercise to lose weight.

We will have food cravings, sugar cravings; we will want junk food and sugary drinks. No one is immune. Those people for whom it seems so easy to stay a healthy weight, they get them too. The first step in losing weight is convincing yourself that you can do this. Let essential oils help you calm your mind and set your foot on the right path to reaching your desired weight or health goals.

How To Use Sandalwood Oil?

Mixing virgin olive oil or coconut oil with essential oils is very common, and you can do this with sandalwood oil as well. Diffuse it and inhale vapors. Make a mixture of 1 drop of sandalwood essential oil and one drop of carrier oil (olive/coconut). Enjoy this aromatherapy and soothe your mind.

Another way to get the best of this essential oil is to rub it directly on your stomach or feet. By rubbing it, you are helping the active compounds of the oil get faster to your cells. You can even consume it: add one or two drops in 1 teaspoon of honey and 4 oz. of coconut milk. Whatever way you chose to use this essential oil, you will feel the benefits and understand why people have used it for thousands of years.

Chapter 8

Fennel Oil

Fennel oil is earthy and sweet and another essential oil that can help deal with weight loss and digestion problems. Besides improving the digestion and suppressing appetite, fennel essential oil provides more restful sleep. Fennel is a source of melatonin, so it helps you get your sleeping cycle right.

Why is sleeping so important for weight loss?

At night, our body has to regenerate and to regenerate properly; we have to get enough of sleep and the right kind of sleep - restful sleep. When we are sleeping, our bodily functions are set to minimum, in order to save energy and to refresh. Our cells regenerate, and our muscles relax. Waking up during the night disturbs our cycle of sleep and interrupts our process of regeneration; our brain is alert again, and we will need extra time to get back to the phase when our body is completely relaxed. People have more and more problems with sleeping these days because of the smartphones, notebooks, IPads and other electronics they bring to bed with them, or they keep with them in their bedroom. Using electronics before going to bed harms our sleep and our brain activity during the night. Electronics have electromagnetic waves, and they radiate. Our body can feel this radiation although we can't see it or feel it ourselves, and these waves are disturbing our sleep rhythms in ways that science is still discovering. In order to have good quality sleep, it's crucial that 15 or even 30 minutes before going to bed is spent relaxing without these devices, (including your kindle - sorry) being used or even near you.

You can meditate, you can do breathing exercises or you can simply inhale diffused essential oils. This time before going to bed is when you calm your mind, silence your thoughts and prepare for a great nights slumber. We've all had situations when we couldn't fall asleep due to problems and thoughts running through our heads for hours. This can create a vicious cycle in which our days are less productive so we can't get anything done and we worry about how we are going to get everything done so now we can't sleep again and it starts again the next day. Leave problems outside your bedroom if you want to wake up with your energy refilled. Use different essential oils for relaxation: inhale them, rub them on your skin or drip a few drops in your warm bath.

Using essential oils like fennel help you get the sleep you need so that you are more productive and can make better decisions. Fennel is a sweet lullaby that helps you have the best sleep of your life every single night.

How To Use Fennel Oil?

Inhale fennel essential oil diluted or make a mixture of 80 drops of fennel, 40 drops of bergamot, and 24 drops of patchouli oil and massage it on abdomen for appetite suppression.

In your produce isle, fennel is that plant that looks a little like celery stalks with a feathery top that looks like the trees from the children's book, and related movies, The Lorax. Fennel stalks are also tasty to eat raw or cooked, and they are highly nutritious. They are used in many Mediterranean cuisines, which are known to be some of the healthiest in the world. Fennel has a subtle sweet licorice taste. But I only recommend that you eat fennel in season because otherwise it has a bitter and rotten taste and if you try it or tried it out of season you may think you don't like it. That is why essential oils are so great. You can get the benefits all year round; because when essential oils are created the benefits are preserved for months or even years to come.

Chapter 9

Lavender Oil

Lavender is another of the oils in use for thousands of years. It is used for culinary purposes as well as in health and beauty purposes. Lavender is often found in perfumes because it gives a very strong base for other scents. Lavender comes from the word "Lavare" (Italian) and it means, "to wash". This plant got its name thanks to the amazing aroma of the flowers, which smell, clean, fresh and vibrant.

Lavender is best known for calming effects. It has a strong relaxing scent that helps us release any stress in no time. It's widely used for treating depression, migraines, headaches, emotional stress, etc. Scientists have thoroughly researched this wonderful plant, so the results are highly supported by strong scientific data: lavender has a huge impact on the autonomic nervous system and because of this asset; lavender is used to treat insomnia and to stabilize heart rate. Researches also show it even boosts cognitive functions, it fights anxiety and it is highly effective in decreasing mental stress.

Weight gain has a lot to do with stress and sleep, as we have mentioned above, so lavender oil can help you to cope with stress and release built up tension in your body. Modern studies have shown that lavender shows better results when fighting insomnia than medicines again and again and again. People keep re-doing the studies. It is like some just can't believe how well it works and that it is that much better than leading prescription sleep aids, which often force your body into sleep mode leaving you feeling groggy the next day. If you ever watched the Wizard of Oz with Judy Garland, you remember the poppy field where everyone wanted to fall asleep. If they had really thought that through, they would have used a lavender field as that would have been much more believable. There are actually whole fields of these beautiful purple flowers on hillsides in Italy and Spain. You should look it up.

Lavender is used to help treat irritation and inflammation throughout the body. When you are trying to lose weight, any inflammation in your body will prevent weight loss because our body is distracted by these "emergencies". Our bodies can be like team supervisors sometimes. If you have ever been a team lead, supervisor or manager, you will absolutely get this reference. They are rushing around, trying to put out fires to the point that they cannot get any work done. These fires in a business are normally caused by bad oversight, planning and prioritizing. It is the same thing with our bodies. Poor planning and choices on our part lead to fires (inflammation) and when or bodies are busy with fires all day long, they cannot work efficiently to burn fat and give us the energy we need to get things done. Using lavender essential oil can help you first, by improving your health, and then you can focus more on losing pounds.

Another benefit of using lavender essential oil is solving respiratory problems. Any throat infections, problems with breathing, coughing, asthma, etc. can make losing weight harder because you are not breathing properly and there is not enough oxygen in your blood to supply the cells. Breathing properly is crucial because our body needs oxygen to function at its best, and if we breathe shallow, it is like driving a car with half-deflated tires. You are wasting a lot of gas and you are wearing your tires out at the same time. Lavender essential oil can help you with respiratory problems and it can improve your breathing capacity.

Lavender helps with mobility of food in the intestine and it promotes production of gastric juices and bile, helping your indigestion and stomach/intestine problems such as gas, diarrhea, flatulence and vomiting. As we have already discussed, when our digestive system is working, as it should, we can absorb nutrients and lose weight.

How To Use Lavender Oil?

Since lavender helps with so many problems, there are many ways to use it. If you have respiratory problems, inhale the vapor of lavender essential oil or rub a few drops on your abdomen. For insomnia problems put a few drops on your pillow, or leave a diffuser with lavender oil in your bedroom. If you have problems with digestion, add a few drops to a glass of water and drink it daily.

Chapter 10

Tangerine Oil

Tangerine is a citrus with a high level of D-limonene, and it is not widely used, since the benefits are still being discovered, but this sweet fruit has a lot to give. Tangerine oil is like that new guy at work who you are not so sure about yet because he hasn't proven himself, but he's a go getter and it won't be long before he is showing you, your boss and the company everything he's got.

Tangerine is so beneficial for the immune system, skin and it is a great digestive aid. Tangerine oil is considered to be a suitable replacement for grapefruit oil. As an excellent source of antioxidants, this oil can be used for total body cleansing and detoxifying. Experts for essential oils say you should change the oils you use every or every second day, so that your body does not become too accustomed to one oil at which point it becomes less effective. We have all seen this happen with shampoo, deodorant, and even exercise. After a while what was once tried and true stops working. Our bodies respond best to variety and that is why it is so great that there are so many oils that have similar effects on our body and mind. But these compounds also have great benefits when they are put together. So, if you are looking for the best option for detoxifying at least once a week combine Grapefruit, Lemon, Tangerine, Mandarin and Lemongrass essential oils to give your body a supercharge. They are all citruses and have similar compounds, but together they will have an amazing result.

Tangerine is also very efficient as a relaxant. It is used for various perfumes and as a natural fragrance in many beauty products.

How To Use Tangerine Oil?

You can add drops in your lemonade, tea or in plain water. For instant energy boost and mood improvement, you can rub a few drops between your palms and inhale from here. It is perfect for making scented candles because the smell is not too strong and it is amazingly relaxing. DIY body scrub is also a great idea to improve your circulation and get your skin free of dead cells. Mix 2 cups of brown sugar, ¼ cup of coconut oil and add 10 drops of Tangerine and Spearmint essential oils.

Chapter 11

Oregano Oil

Oregano oil is one of the most powerful cleansing and purifying agents of all essential oils. It has countless benefits and it is a must if you are trying to help your body detox. Wild Oregano oil is also used for fighting Candida (yeast overgrowth) and it is highly anti-bacterial.

It takes a small amount of this strong oil to make a big difference. Oregano oil is used for boosting the immune system, for respiratory support and muscles and joints. Besides these benefits, oregano oil helps healthy digestion, which is crucial for weight loss.

Back to cleansing and purifying. This is crucial, not only for weight loss, but your health in general. If you leave toxins sitting in your body, you could suffer from various inflammations, intestinal problems, digestion problems, etc. With just a few drops of this oil, you can help your body become healthy and toxin-free again.

Be very careful that you are buying wild oregano oil from a reputable company. Just because it smells like oregano, does not mean that the oil has been made with the required potency (strength) to actually do its job. Make note of how many drops are considered a serving size. Some bottles will say as many as 30-40 drops is a serving size, which means you are using half the bottle and it is not strong at all. Others will say that 2-3 is a serving and these are usually made with the correct potency. These bottles can be relatively expensive compared to other oils at around $35 for 1 ounce (around 100 drops), but if you have to use 40 drops (almost half the bottle) of the cheap one to see any results, have you saved any money by buying the cheap one? In the long run, no you haven't.

How To Use Oregano Oil?

Yes, you can put a few drops on your pasta, pizza or in spaghetti sauce. It has the same taste as the oregano we eat, just a lot stronger. It is the concentrate of the oregano we eat, just like every essential oil is the concentrate of a plant or fruit. You should be careful with applying it on your skin because this is a hot oil, that actually burns when a concentrated amount is left on the skin, so it should be diluted with some other oils (coconut or extra virgin olive oil) before use. And if you just applying a drop or two in your mouth on the run, be sure to drink a glass of water after to avoid the burning effects if it sits on your teeth, gums and tongue. Some brands recommend leaving under tongue for up to a minute to absorb. This is alright as the burn effect is slow, but you will feel a burning sensation, which will be pronounced the first time you use it, so don't get caught off guard. Adding a drop or two of oregano oil to a glass of water during cold and flu season can be a safe alternative and help bolster your immune system while helping to detox your body. If you know or suspect you have an infection, such as a bladder infection, some research has shown that oil of oregano can knock it out, but only if taken in higher quantities than you would take for maintenance. However, never delay seeking medical treatment for serious infections if symptoms have not significantly improved in 2-3 days, because some infections can be life threatening and in the case of a really bad bladder infection it can move into your kidneys, which could be really bad news. I really dislike prescribed antibiotics because of their side effects, like Candida overgrowth and antibiotic resistant bacteria, but if your infection is severe, sometimes Rx's are the only thing that will work since essential oils work in a slow and measured way that may not be able to catch up with an infection that is already out of the ballpark. Make essential oil use a part of your daily routine and they really should limit If not eliminate the need for more conventional treatment methods in a lot of cases.

Chapter 12

Spearmint Oil

You've come across spearmint in toothpaste, candies or chewing gums. It is widely in use for adding flavor, but spearmint has many therapeutic uses as well. It is great support for the digestive system and immune system. Spearmint oil can aid in digestion, meaning it can contribute to your weight loss, and it can help with occasional stomachaches. Spearmint has a carminative effect as well, helping the gasses in the stomach and intestines to pass out of the body naturally without causing a lot of unnecessary pain and bloatedness. When your stomach and intestine are relaxed and pain relieved, your body can focus on fat burning. Maybe the most important role of spearmint is it's stimulant effects. Spearmint stimulates the secretion of hormones, gastric juices and bile and it boosts your metabolism to burn more fat. Having proper blood circulation is important for weight loss because if there's poor circulation, our cells won't get enough oxygen, and this could leave our bodies depleted of necessary vitamins and minerals.

Spearmint has shown great results in helping with constipation and excess flatulence. When trying to lose weight, we are trying to keep our metabolic activity on a high rate, meaning our body needs to get rid of toxins and excess fat from our body. Slow metabolism will slow weight loss and constipation can lead to many serious problems if not treated. Improving diet while incorporating spearmint oil can be the perfect arsenal to kick start long-term weight loss.

How To Use Spearmint Oil?

Make a craving curber diffuser blend: mix 3 drops of grapefruit oil, 3 drops of lemon oil and 1 drop of spearmint oil

Add a few drops to your morning glass of water, rub a few drops on palms and inhale for respiration problems. For promoting digestion, add a few drops to your desserts, drinks, salads, etc. You can use it daily in your tea and help prevent digestion problems and reduce stress.

Conclusion

All the oils discussed can be made at home by simply growing an herb or flower garden of your choice and harvesting them for your oils. However, most choose to take the quickest most efficient route and that is buying them from your local health and nutrition store. I feel acquiring the oils is the easy part, actually making the decision to start taking them and incorporating them into your daily routine is the part that most will struggle with.

Your body and mind are the most important things in your life. Even if you are a person who always puts others first, you can only be there for those you love, doing the things you love, if you are nurturing your body and mind.

Losing weight is easy if you starve yourself, but then as soon as you can't take it anymore, you are likely going to rebound and gain it all back and likely a lot more. Each time we "yo-yo" we make it harder and harder to lose weight and easier to gain it all back. Being the ideal weight is never healthy if you achieve it in an unhealthy way like starving, using artificial stimulants or working out 8 hours a day (yes it happens). People who do these things may love what they see when they step on the scale in the morning, but those results are often short lived. What I've presented in this book isn't some hocus pocus spell for overnight success, but my hope is that the things that I've shared with you can shed some light on essential oils and open your eyes to possibilities maybe you've never considered before.

My hope is that maybe you can stop feeling tired and stop feeling depressed. Stop accepting that stress, pain and poor health is just a part of life, just a part of getting older. It's not. Stop letting your cravings rule your life by telling you what to eat and when to eat instead of letting your mind make good choices for you that will make you feel better in the long run. Your cravings may not even be "your" cravings if your body is not in balance.

A side note of advice; once you start losing the weight and feeling amazing, don't be afraid to try new things. Go on a day hike or learn how to salsa dance, do those things that you've only thought about doing in the past, take action. One other thing I encourage you to do is share your experience with those around you. Gifts are best when given away, and if these oils prove to be a gift in what they add to your life, than please let those around you and those you care about in on the secret so they too can experience the joy and fullness that you now feel.

Never forget that a strong body is best achieved and maintained with a strong mind and in order to lose weight you need to be at peace with yourself and find balance in life. Essential oils are amazing when used properly and are used as a full body approach to overall well-being, and can truly make a positive impact on your present and future life. So I urge and implore you to explore the wonderful world of nature and what it's given us, and let it help you become a better, healthier version of you. You deserve it!!

Thank you so much for purchasing my book!! If you enjoyed it at all I would be forever grateful if you would leave me a review on Amazon.com

All the best!!

www.ingramcontent.com/pod-product-compliance
Lightning Source LLC
Chambersburg PA
CBHW072022290526
45787CB00013B/1738